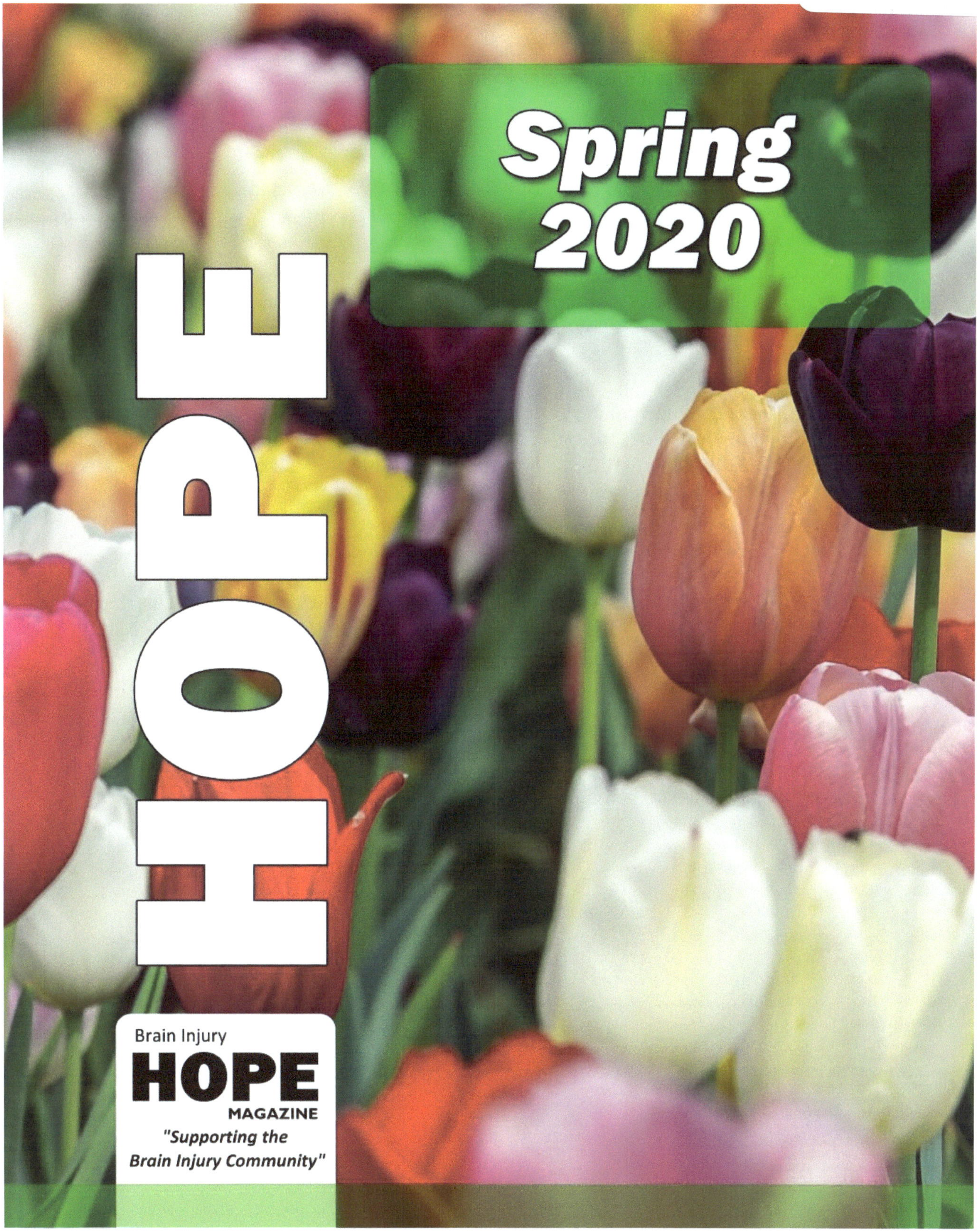

Spring
2020

HOPE

Brain Injury
HOPE
MAGAZINE
"Supporting the
Brain Injury Community"

Welcome

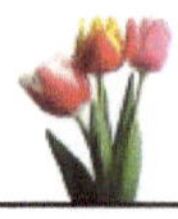

HOPE MAGAZINE

Serving the Brain Injury Community Since 2015

Spring 2021

Publisher
David A. Grant

Editor
Sarah Grant

Our Contributors

Linda M. Ansell
Andrew Davie
David A. Grant
Sarah Grant
Sarah Jackson
Ric Johnson
James Scott
Rebecca Veenstra

Welcome to the Spring 2021 Issue of HOPE Magazine

March is an exciting month in the brain injury community as we come together to celebrate Brain Injury Awareness Month here in the United States.

And why not call it a celebration? It's a month where advocacy becomes front and center. Awareness events dot the landscape both locally and nationally. Survivors have the opportunity to come together (at least virtually), and for a short time, brain injury is talked about more than the remaining eleven months of the year.

But we still live in the shadow of 2020. The last year has been one of unfathomable loss. To try to wrap words around the degree of loss our shared humanity has experienced would not even scratch the surface. But 2021 has a good dose of something we did not have last year – hope!

As we move deeper into this year, life may start to look a bit more like it used to. My "hope" for you is that you will come away from this month's issue feeling that you are perhaps a little less alone in your journey, and that there are others who share your fate, and who have found a way to build meaningful lives after brain injury.

Peace,

David A. Grant
Publisher

Table
of Contents

02 Publisher's Introduction

04 Becoming a Different Me

08 Stay Strong, Stay Safe

11 Education Equals Rehabilitation

14 A Caregiver's Perspective

16 Decision Time

19 Comfortably Numb

23 Dear Friend

27 The COVID-19 Wildcard

29 News & Views

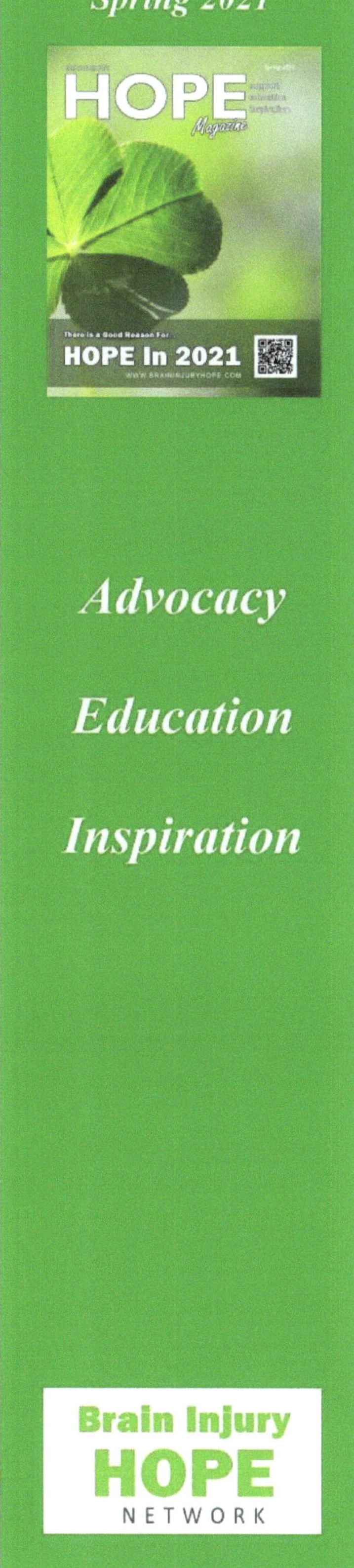

Becoming a Different Me

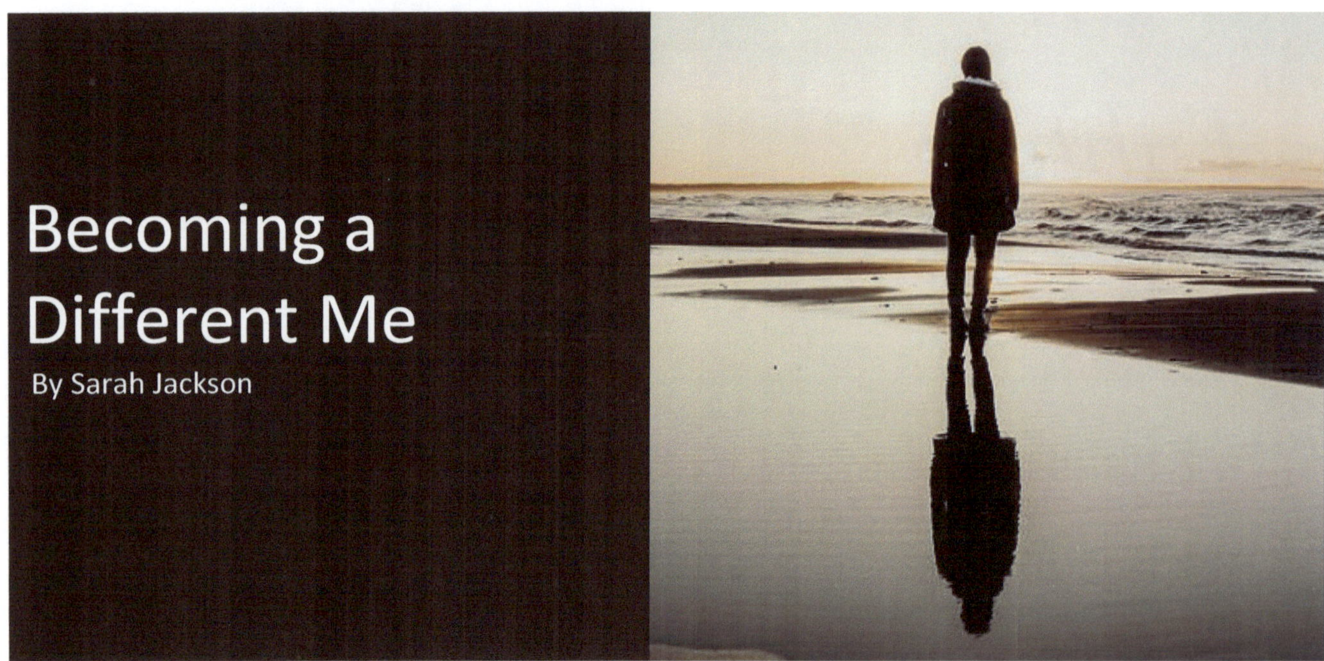

By Sarah Jackson

When I am me, I am always thinking of becoming a different me; yoga me, writer me, dental assistant me (hey, it could happen), workout me, and even the better mom me. However, the truth is that while I'm spending so much time thinking of where I want to be, and who I want to be, that I'm ignoring the essence of who I should be, and that is the real me. The problem is that I am not present where I am. I would like to come to terms with a reality I can accept.

Except that can't happen, especially on days when my brain is struggling to make it out of the grocery story. The grocery store dilemma is a common one for me. My husband asked me to get the milk, cereal, and eggs. There were only three items on my list. While this sounds easy enough, I have a brain injury. "I can memorize those," I thought with a bit of hope. My husband and I then went our separate ways in the grocery store. "Divide and Conquer" as we like to say.

> "After putting the cake in the basket, I start heading down an aisle filled with bright colors, candies, and decorations. And why not? A lot of people are in the aisle so surely I must need something there too."

The trouble is that I get distracted somewhere between produce and dairy. I find myself in the bread aisle picking out enticing cake flavors and frosting colors. I am suddenly overwhelmed with the many options available that I decide buying one from the bakery section of the store would be a better choice. Quickly won over by the Coconut Macaroon cake in the freezer, I tell my brain to refocus and get what I came for – something so easy for those without an injury. After putting the cake in the basket, I start heading down an aisle filled with bright colors, candies, and decorations. And why not? A lot of people are in the aisle so surely I must need something there too. It made 100% sense at the time.

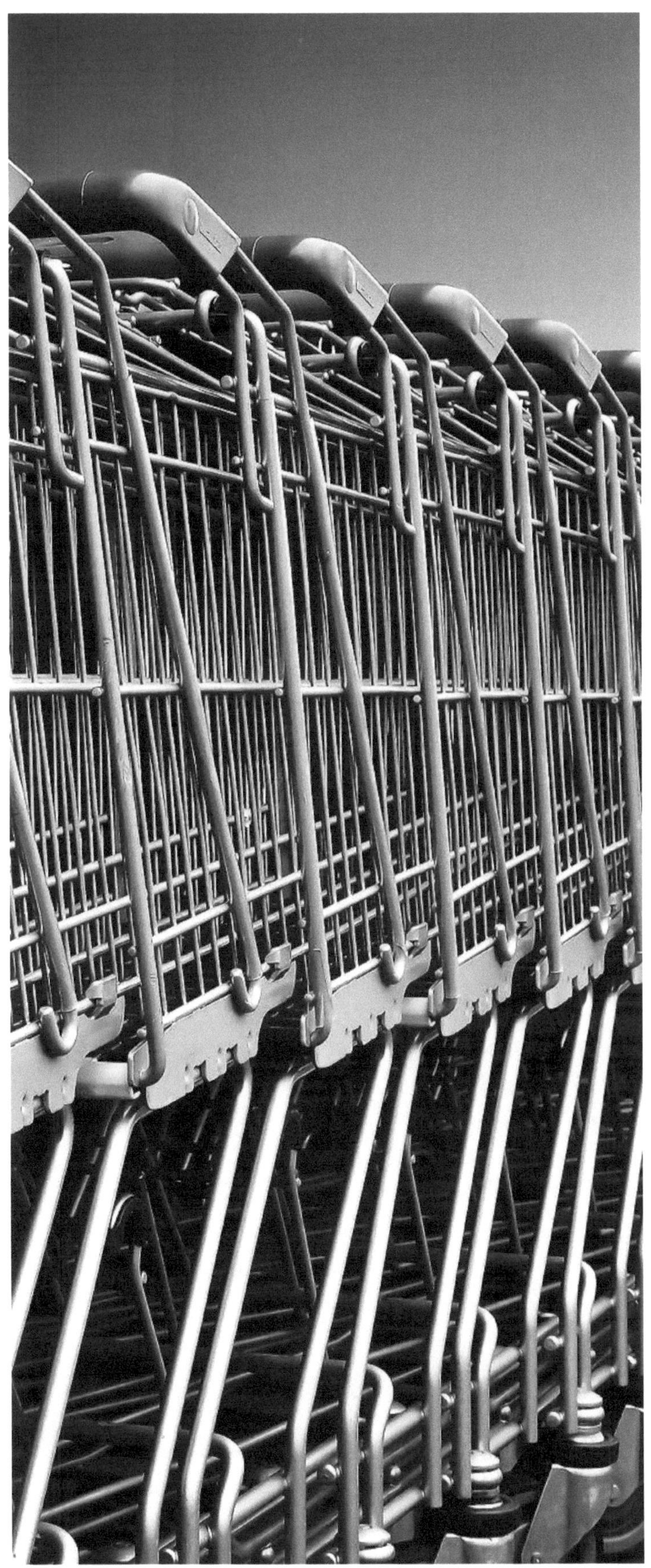

After perusing the section, I grab what my kids would like best and finally make it to the milk section. Bombarded with varieties and prices and thoughts of other activities to be done that day, I feel myself emotionally begin to erupt with anxiety and tension that I wasn't expecting. Remember, I only needed to get three things.

"You know what? I'll just grab one of each and let him decide. But first, I need a cart with wheels in order to accomplish this mission." While making my way to the entrance where the carts sit, I see a vacant cart ahead. I load the cake into the cart. Astonishingly, a woman comes toward me. "Hey, that's my cart!" she announces, clearly annoyed with me. For goodness' sake, get me out of here. I don't like this feeling and clearly, I don't belong here.

As if a war over grocery carts were about to take place, I immediately removed my hands from the shopping cart and excuse myself for making such a rash decision. Grabbing the cake, I continue to the front of the store, making sure no one is using the next cart I have my eyes on. Not wanting another cart war to break out, I quickly grab it and head back to the dairy aisle. 'Okay, I have a cart," I say under my breath as if I'm about to run out of oxygen.

Keeping myself together, remembering the task now is to load each of the six varieties of milk he may be talking about, I start filling the cart. Before I knew it, my cart contained skim milk, whole milk (because it's on sale,) 1% milk because I like it, 2% milk because the kids like it, soy unsweetened milk because he's on a diet and soy sweetened milk because it tastes like a milkshake and I will need one when I am finished here.

Remembering I was told to get the cereal, because cereal is the perfect companion for milk, I head toward the cereal aisle. The thing I love about the cereal aisle is that you cannot miss it - it's the whole aisle. The problem now is that there are so many to choose from. I don't know what, or where to get the cereal he mentioned. Instead of freaking out, I calm myself and grab the most expensive and interesting kind of cereal I've ever heard of. My reasoning made sense at the time: it sounds good, and I've never tried it.

At this point, I'm feeling completely emotionally run-down and overly embarrassed from my shopping cart episode. Wanting to cover my face with my hands and let the tears flow, I decide now is not the place to do so.

After retracing the aisles several times in search of my husband, I finally spot him in the corner of my eye. Forgetting that I am not the Energizer Bunny I used to be, I suddenly feel incompetent to even maneuver something as simple as grocery shopping. Clearly now completely out of energy, and emotionally drained from my shopping experience, my first thought is to blame my husband for such an ordeal.

If it wasn't for him delegating this not-so-easy task for me, I wouldn't be in such a crazed mess. But I am overly-exhausted now. This trip through the grocery store has required enough energy to last all weekend.

But it's not his fault. It's nobody's fault. I wanted to help. I am me and clearly, I cannot accept me.

Apparently, there is a threshold for people like me. It's called resistance and it happens each morning the alarm goes off. Not wanting to give up, or to give in to challenges ahead, we will awake to and confront the battles before us. Very much wanting to overlook our difficulties and combat our struggles, we know the process is a far reach. At the end of the day though, we know we have made it thus far, and can only appreciate the resilience required to get here. Look far into the distance, what do you see? You can be imperfect. You can make mistakes. Better still, you just can be you.

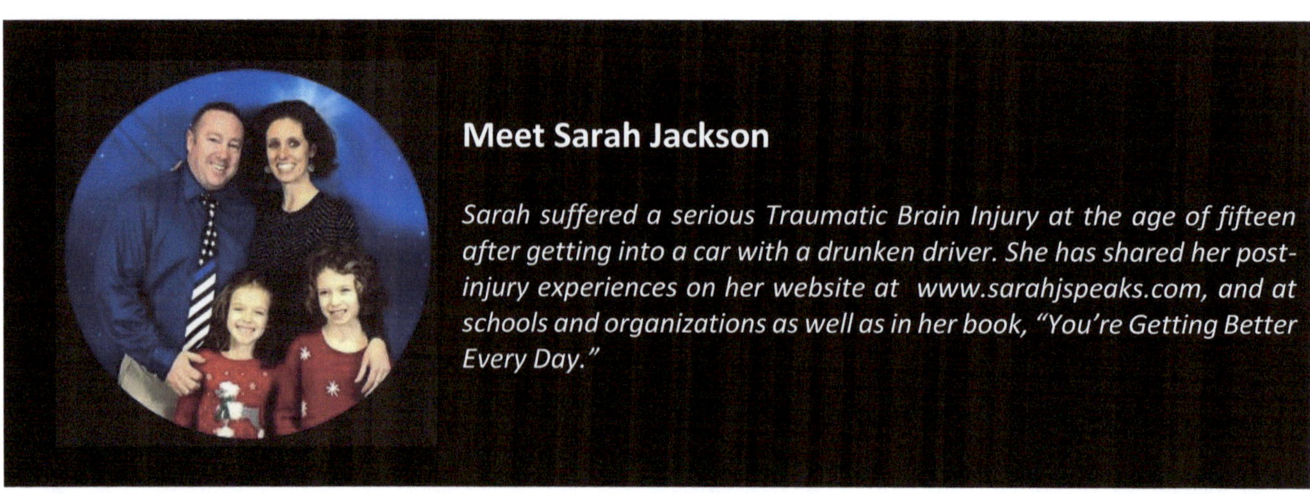

Meet Sarah Jackson

Sarah suffered a serious Traumatic Brain Injury at the age of fifteen after getting into a car with a drunken driver. She has shared her post-injury experiences on her website at www.sarahjspeaks.com, and at schools and organizations as well as in her book, "You're Getting Better Every Day."

Contributors Wanted!

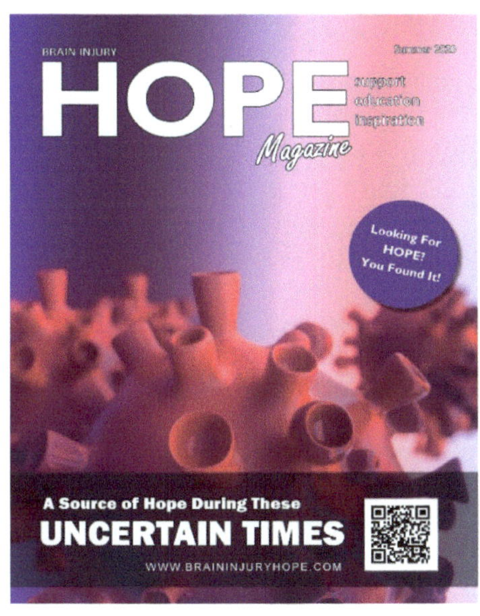

Got A Story To Tell?

We are accepting stories for the Summer 2021 issue of HOPE Magazine!

Your story has the power to help others.

The Summer 2021 issue of HOPE Magazine will be available in June.

Your Story has Value!

And now the details...

- We prefer an article length of 800-1,000 words. Longer or shorter pieces will be considered.
- When submitting, please include a photo and short bioto be included with your piece.

Please email your submission to info@tbihopeandinspiration.com.

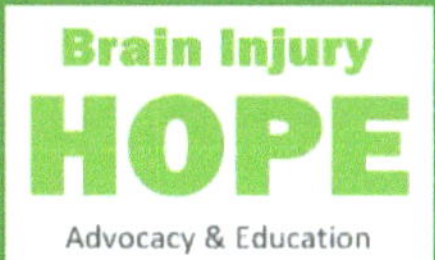

Stay Strong, Stay Safe

By Ric Johnson

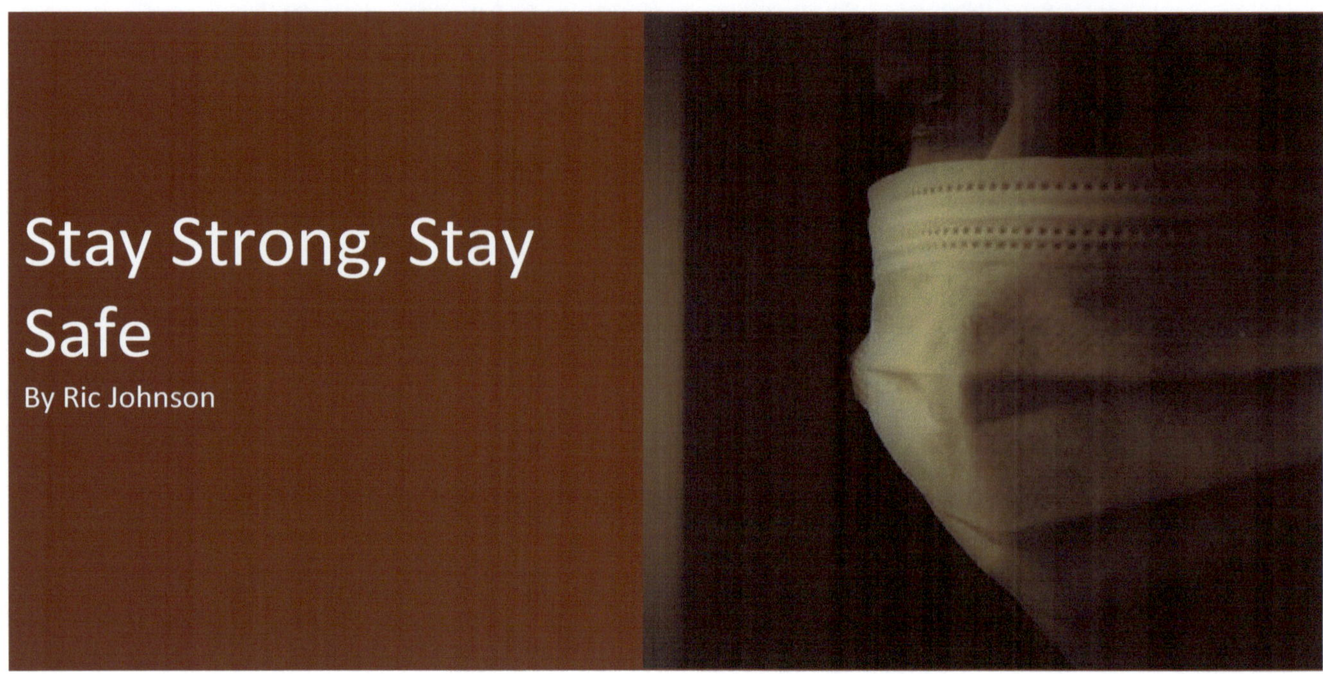

Over seventeen years ago I fell off a ladder while cleaning the gutters on my house. I awoke thirty days later and started my very own quarantine. While I wasn't really alone, I was isolated from others because of my craniology surgery, so it felt like I was alone. I saw my wife for an hour in the evenings, my kids a few hours on weekends, and my brother and sister when they had time. At least, that's what I remember.

I've been told that at least one of my family members was at my side for many hours, virtually every day. During the first ninety days, after waking up from a medically induced coma, I was transferred to three hospitals for speech, physical, and occupation therapy. I had to re-learn everything I knew before I started grade school. Only then, I went back home.

> "During the first ninety days, after waking up from a medically induced coma, I was transferred to three hospitals for speech, physical, and occupation therapy."

At the time I couldn't drive so I had family, or friends, drive me to therapy sessions or doctor appointments. I could not do much of anything physically or mentally either. Except for my helpers, I was alone. I learned how to believe in myself. I learned the difference between being physically or mentally fatigued and the difference between waiting and accepting as well as the difference between before and now.

I retired from my job in February 2020 thinking that being a retired senior citizen will be great fun, a life I could handle even with aphasia, short term memory, but most importantly, without stress. Boy was I wrong. In March of 2020 my city, my state, the USA and pretty much the whole world shut down. Right away it wasn't too hard, maybe odd, but still okay.

COVID-19 pandemic was like a kick in the gut. The governor of Minnesota proclaimed a Stay at Home order with the social distancing edict. It felt almost the same as my first year as a traumatic brain injury survivor. During that first year after my TBI, I wasn't stopped to do much, and I needed more help. But now? Everything is changed. I'm unable to see my grandkids, unable to have meals with my friends or at a restaurant, and unable to go shopping; I'm unable to go to my local library and browse the shelves. I'm unable to go and see anything that catches my eye or mind. I refuse to call this the "new normal." I already went through the new normal phase in 2004.

At my age (71) I think *This Too Shall Pass* is such a great phrase. I just hope it doesn't take too much time to achieve. But until then, it is up to me to live my life as fully as possible. To that end I have found that adapting seems to be the key. I also discovered that being outside is better than inside. Instead of binge watching the TV, I walk to the garden and sit at the patio to look and listen to the birds. I often find a digital book to read or re-read an old book I find in the house. Sometimes I just watch the clouds.

Thinking about things that I can't do, only makes the pandemic worst. Whenever I feel stuck, or out-of-whack, moving is another key. Maybe the weather makes me stay inside but I can still get up and walk to another room just to see if everything is in its place. If I see a neighbor outside, I can go out to say

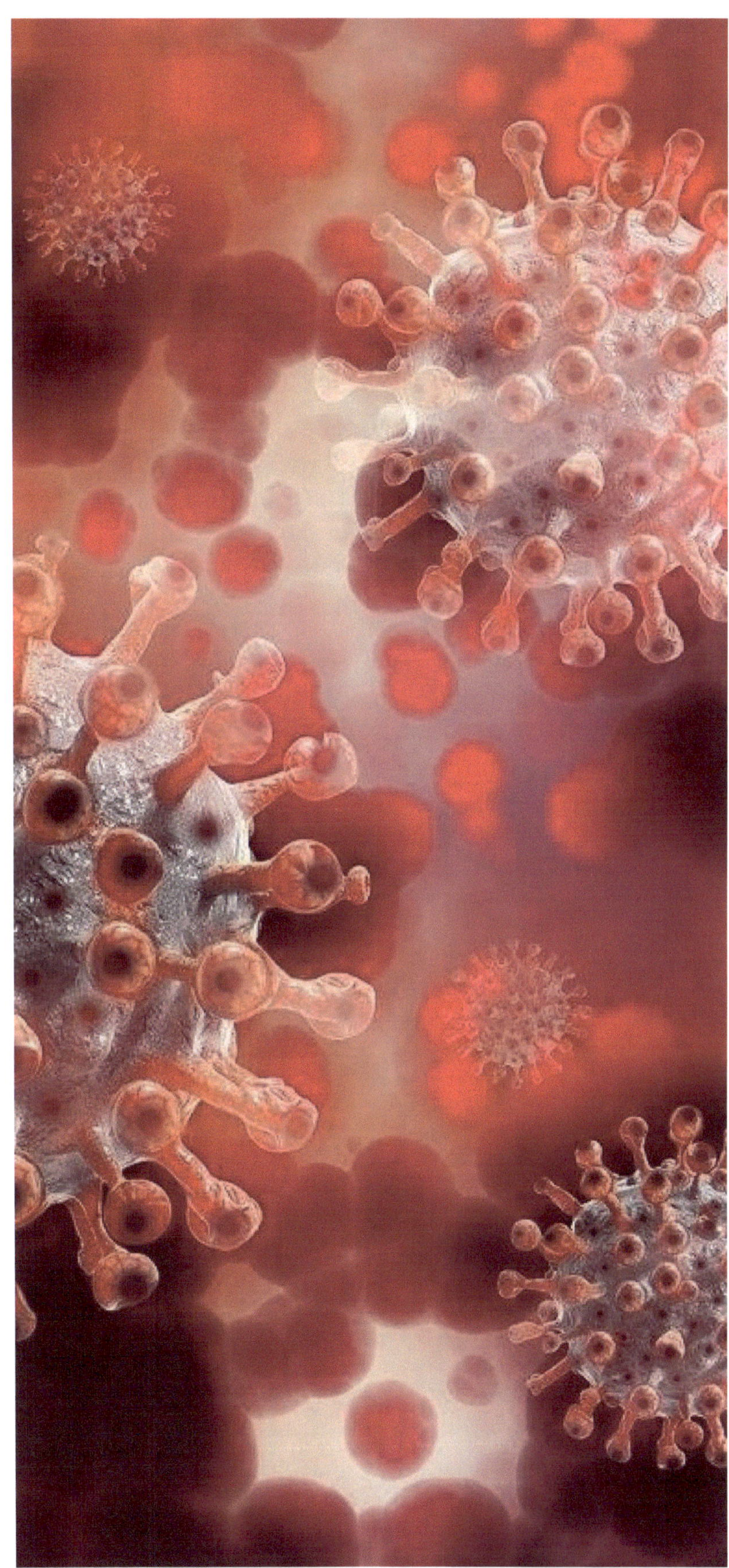

hello. I can play a record, sing along with the band and dance - especially if my wife isn't watching.

Staying at home doesn't mean I'm totally cut off from the world, I just need to make sure to stay in contact with others who are also staying home. I call friends or family members just to say hello. I only know a few phone numbers from members of the support group I attend, so I try to call them as well. I also post a message on the support groups Facebook page at least once a month.

Pandemic is a word I probably never said before, probably was not even able to spell it, but pandemic is a word I know way too much at this time. I know that if I get sick everything changes, so I have to make sure that is not going to happen. How can I make sure? Until I and others have been vaccinated, I need to live in my own state of mind, under my control, as well as I can.

Does that mean I've given up? Not even close. It means I believe in science. During these last twelve months, I make sure to leave my house only when it absolutely necessary. Instead of shopping in my grocery store I order groceries online and use their pick-up services when they tell me it's ready. When I'm in a public area, I have used every way I know to keep moving forward: wearing a face mask; wearing gloves; keeping six feet away; washing my hands and using a hand sanitizer.

It does seem, at times, that whatever I want to do contradicts what I need to do. I lived through a traumatic brain injury and made my family live though my recovery process. That is the last thing I want to go through again. So, I hold my breath, and follow the rules that gives me hope that COVID-19 will not lead my life forever. Stay Strong, Stay Safe.

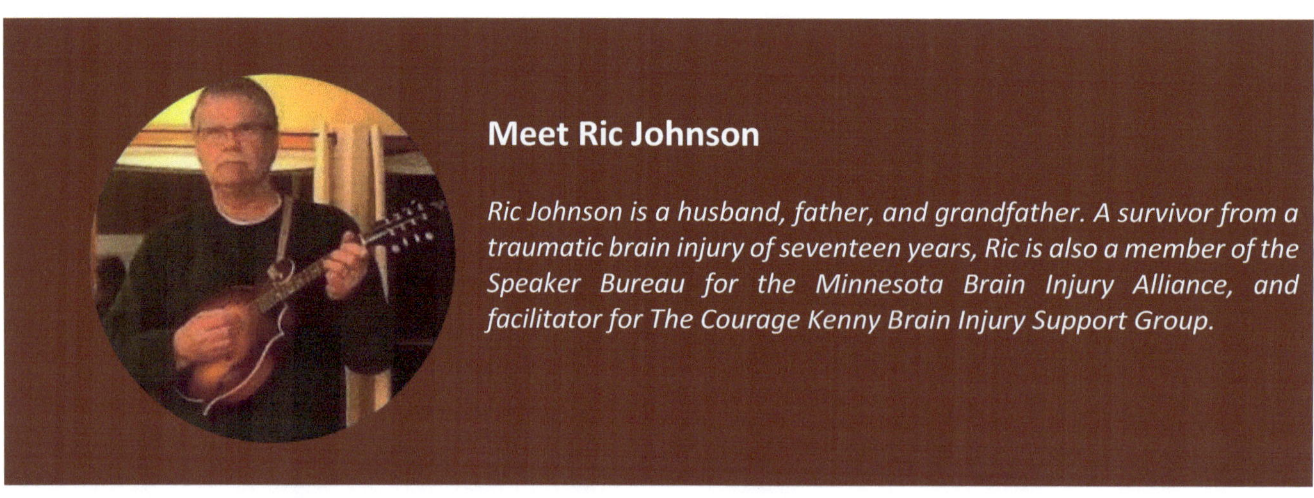

Meet Ric Johnson

Ric Johnson is a husband, father, and grandfather. A survivor from a traumatic brain injury of seventeen years, Ric is also a member of the Speaker Bureau for the Minnesota Brain Injury Alliance, and facilitator for The Courage Kenny Brain Injury Support Group.

Perseverance is failing 19 times and succeeding the 20th.

-Julie Andrews

Education Equals Rehabilitation

By Lisa M. Ansell

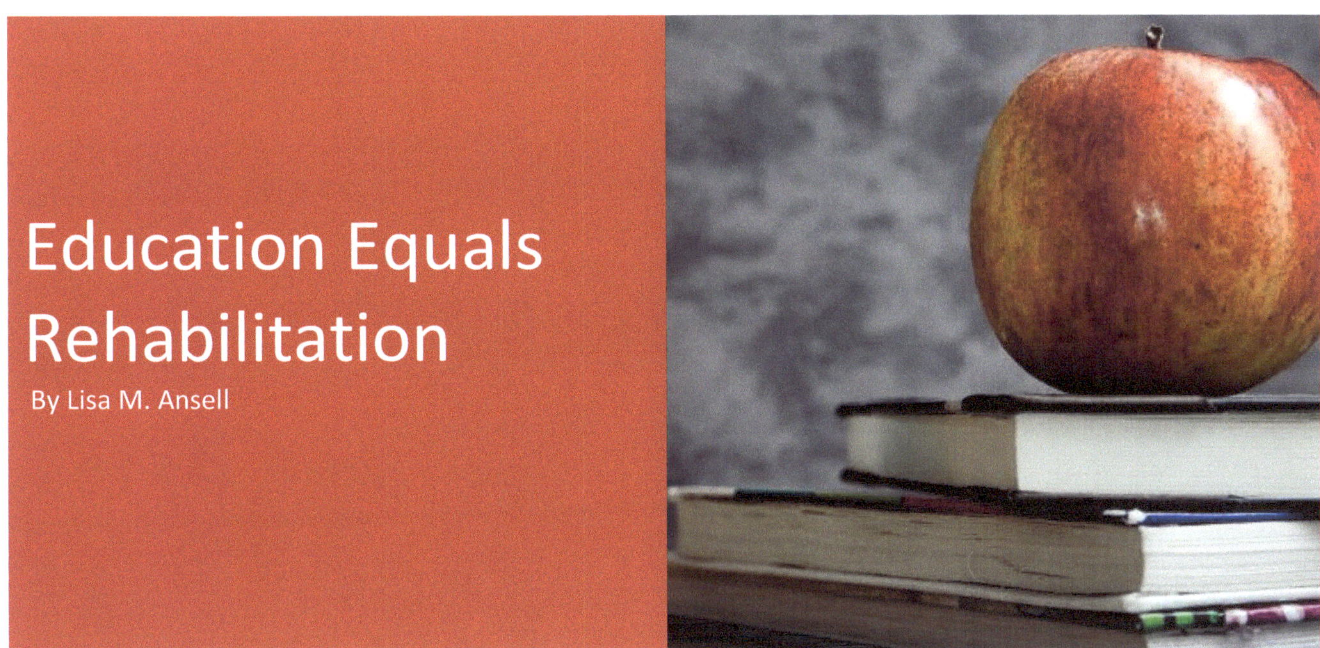

I survived a car accident in 2008, where I was diagnosed with a mild TBI. After the accident, I struggled with memory and word recollection issues, and my relationships began to diminish, one by one. I lived in a rural community where physical and mental health care choices were limited, at best. Oddly, I could remember how I use to be and who I was, but I no longer had the ability to be that person anymore.

My frustration and anger seeped inside of me like a steeping teabag in scolding water. People labeled me "different, awkward, and weird." I looked fine to them, and they labeled me as they chose, spreading the word that I was a liability due to my injury. The personal injury attorneys who were supposed to look after my best interest told me I would be sitting on the couch collecting social security benefits (I was denied more than once and do not have benefits). Success for my future was not in the cards.

> "My frustration and anger seeped inside of me like a steeping teabag in scolding water. People labeled me 'different, awkward, and weird.'"

Filled with despair and lacking hope, I contemplated ending my life. The world had grown meaner than I had previously known (and it was mean), and people were quick to judge and spread inaccurate information about me and my values. So, I sat at my kitchen table, bowed my head to pray for the courage to end my life, and the strangest thing happened. I was inspired to apply to a university and work toward a degree. Yeah, I heard the lawyers' voices remind me how I would not make it through my first class and probably would not get accepted. I decided to listen to the inspiration and apply. One more rejection before I die was not going to hurt anything.

A couple of weeks after submitting my application, I saw a word that changed my life: "accepted." I was accepted into a university I had heard such wonderful things about and, in my wildest dreams, did not think I would get in.

Where the lack of treatment failed me, education became my rehabilitation. I struggled. I could not remember anything I read and would have to spend hours reading the same chapter repeatedly to get the material into my short-term and long-term memory. Somehow, my brain made adaptations to compensate for my memory struggles, and I began succeeding in my coursework. When I walked across the stage to get my first college degree, I felt like I had shown the naysayers up after graduating with honors. I had issues shaking the university president's hand, but you can only do so much when you are overstimulated. Good and bad.

There have been other degrees since then, but education is more than having expensive paper on the wall. Education is training to serve others.

Today, I am at places I did not think I would be. I have worked hard for every accomplishment, setback, and joy I have experienced. I still struggle with overstimulation, interpersonal relationship issues, and the stigmas associated with invisible disabilities, but I keep trying. However, I have dedicated my career to serving others and the TBI community from a mental health perspective. Getting an education was a hidden blessing from the accident. Am I different? Yes, I try before I quit. I work to succeed, and if you think success comes from a paycheck, then success will always fail to measure up. Am I awkward? Well, people who have not walked in my shoes seem awkward to me, so I guess we are even. Am I weird? Sure. I like to learn from each experience, opportunity, and research.

My message of hope to the TBI community is that the only people who can mentally stop us from understanding our new lives are ourselves. I am stuck with my brain injury, but the brain injury is also stuck with me.

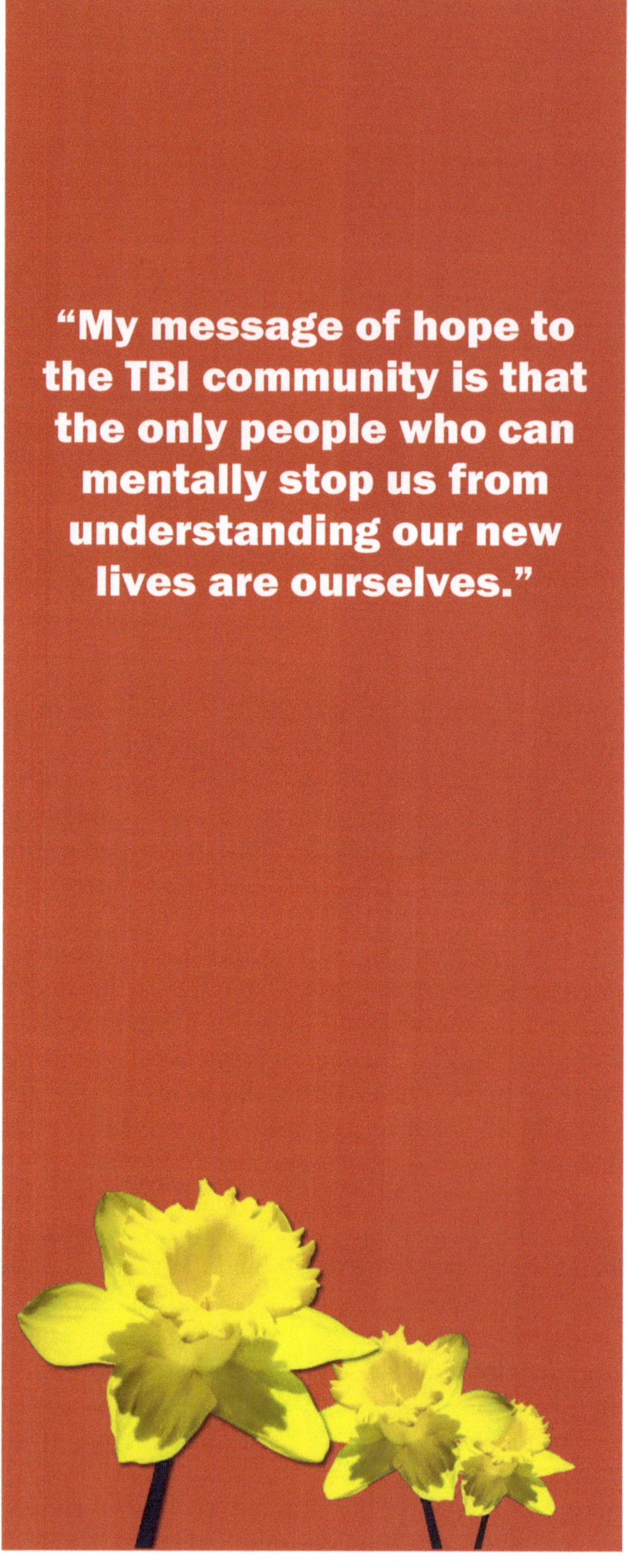

I am more stubborn than the injury will ever be. Although our loved ones can be supportive, we, as survivors, must do the footwork to make positive changes in our lives. The accident showed me who my true friends and loved ones are, and the accident also showed me that I am a lot more than what people think and say about me.

By the grace of God, I have learned to overcome my obstacles instead of being overcome by them. Am I completely accepting of these thoughts? Not every day. However, when I look back to how far I have come and the blessings I have been given in life, and I bow my head to pray, it is not to have the strength to end my life; it is for the strength to be there for others when they walk in the emotional shoes of despair, as I once did. Am I free from emotional despair? Of course not, but I have learned healthier coping skills and ways to filter my thoughts to curb my reactions. It takes time. It takes work. It takes commitment, but we are not alone—reflection, words, and within our shared experiences, there is hope.

Little things mean a lot.

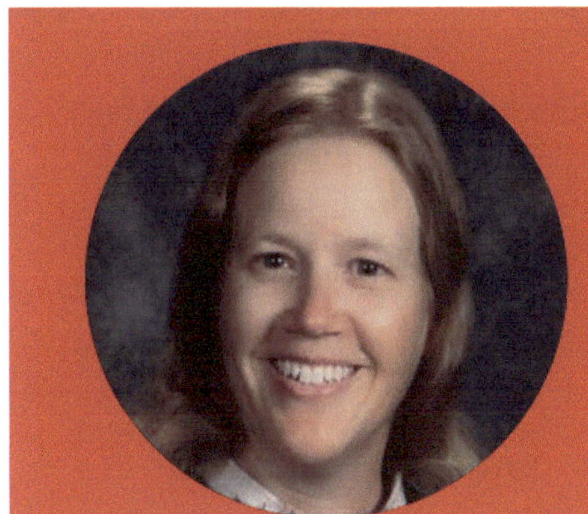

Meet Lisa Ansell

A thirteen year brain injury survivor, Lisa M. Ansell, Ed.D., LPC, NCC, CBIS is a Licensed Professional Counselor, National Certified Counselor, and Certified Brain Injury Specialist. Her hope is that others will be inspired to live their best lives possible after brain injury.

Living With Hope

By Patrick Brigham

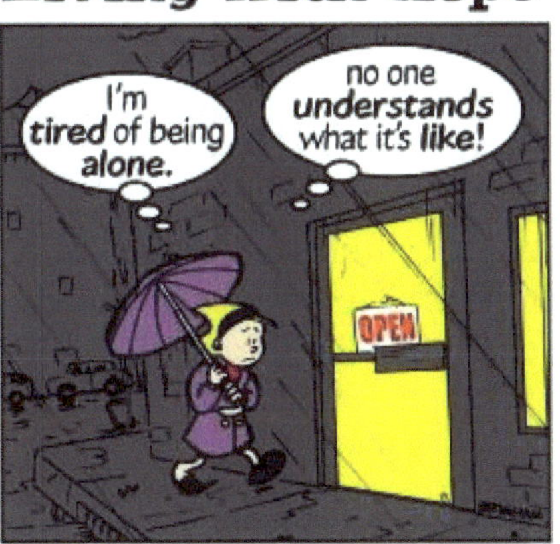

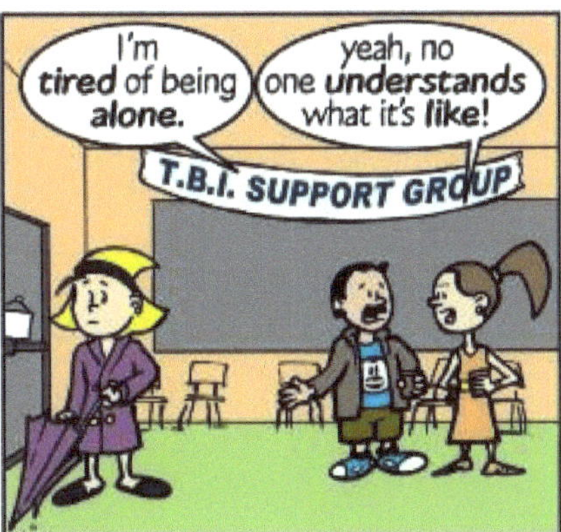

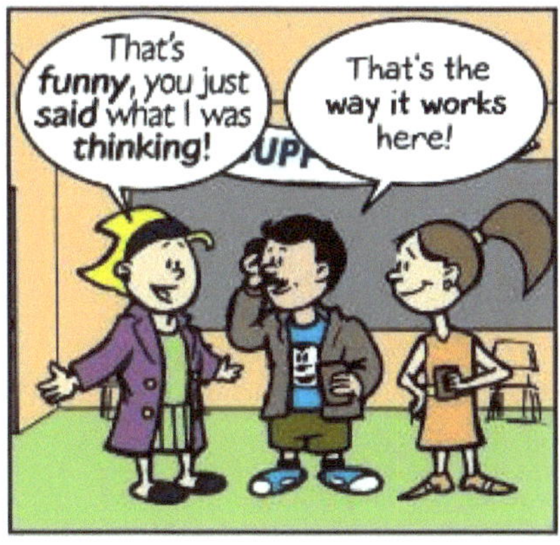

A Caregiver's Perspective

By Sarah Grant

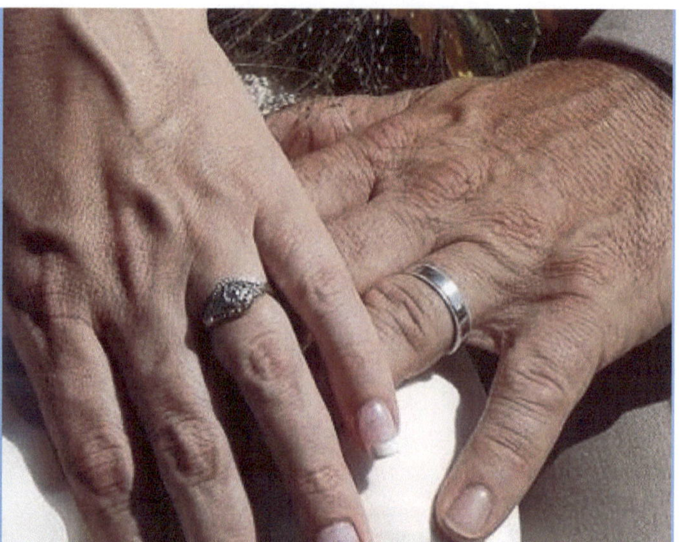

When my husband was injured back in 2010, we were newlyweds with eight children, and we had very full schedules. I'd gone to visit a friend in the hospital while my husband left for his 30-mile daily bicycle ride. Who knew we'd see each other again at the local trauma center? He was hit by a car that Veteran's day, by a teenage schoolmate of our children. As the weeks and months passed after his diagnosis of traumatic brain injury, neither of us suspected that the accident would change us forever.

In the beginning, he suffered from many nightmares and was later diagnosed with PTSD. He had constant ringing in his ears and shook his head a lot as if to cast off the tinnitus that never ceased. He forgot things – so many things, including conversations and appointments. He lost the concept of time, and an hour in the real world only felt like a couple of minutes to him. The passage of time was a big deal when I couldn't reach him, and messages were left unanswered. He was plagued with constant thoughts of suicide and felt that I would be better off without him.

> "Our children were confused and some of them walked away from us and our problems. Friends stopped calling because they felt helpless."

Our children were confused and some of them walked away from us and our problems. Friends stopped calling because they felt helpless. Family members saw us for small windows of time and let us know we looked "fine." At work, my co-workers were concerned about how my husband was doing, but they were also concerned about me. I was tired all the time and I was scattered, in thoughts and in actions.

I initially contacted the Brain Injury Association to locate some support groups nearby that my husband could attend. He needed help coping with his loss of "self" and we thought it would be a good idea to learn everything we could about TBI. We found a local group for survivors only and he flourished there. The members had varying experiences, and lots of compensatory strategies were identified and perfected in their time spent together each month. Suddenly, he had hope.

I wanted hope too!

After about a year, my husband's survivor group was extended to include caregivers. Each month, I looked forward to talking with other spouses about how they kept it all together, and what things worked well in managing their households.

Eventually, the survivors – and specifically MY survivor – didn't want their foibles discussed openly. I stopped attending the support group so he could continue to grow into his new self. I was alone. I considered separating myself from his TBI. The relationship we were in before the accident was kind and loving and mutually supportive; I wanted the best for my husband and our children.

Our relationship after the accident was no longer mutually giving and rewarding; it felt like an obligation and was sometimes one-sided. My personal search for a support group started and ended in one single day: there were no meetings specifically for Caregivers in the entire state of New Hampshire. That had to change! Caregivers are the people who love and support survivors. I didn't want to find out what happened to caregivers who weren't loved and supported.

Our local library agreed to host space for a group meeting each month. I sent emails to all of my friends; I posted flyers around town; I sent an invitation to all of my contacts on Facebook. We had a caregiver group!

Each month, I looked forward to our group meeting. When group members are unable to attend, several of us still talk via email. I've learned that support comes in many ways, and even in giving, I receive. Parents, spouses, and family members have attended the group, and each has contributed a piece of the puzzle that is my life since my husband's accident. I still don't know how many pieces are missing in my personal puzzle, but I do know that getting together to share our common bond helped me feel stronger and more supported.

That caregiver group has long since closed its doors, members got busy living life, and people moved on. But I will always be grateful for the role of peer support in my own personal journey.

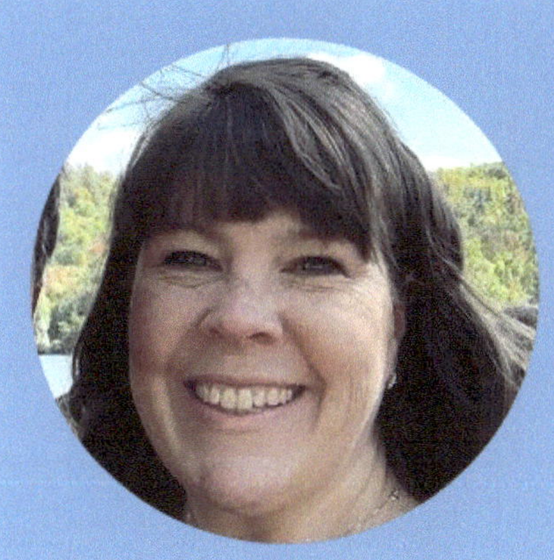

Meet Sarah Grant

*Sarah lives in Salem, NH with her husband and two kittens.
She started an online Caregiver group in 2013, to help make sense of what she was experiencing, and it has grown to almost 7,000 members around the world. She can usually be found outdoors, enjoying life with her husband.*

Decision Time

By James Scott

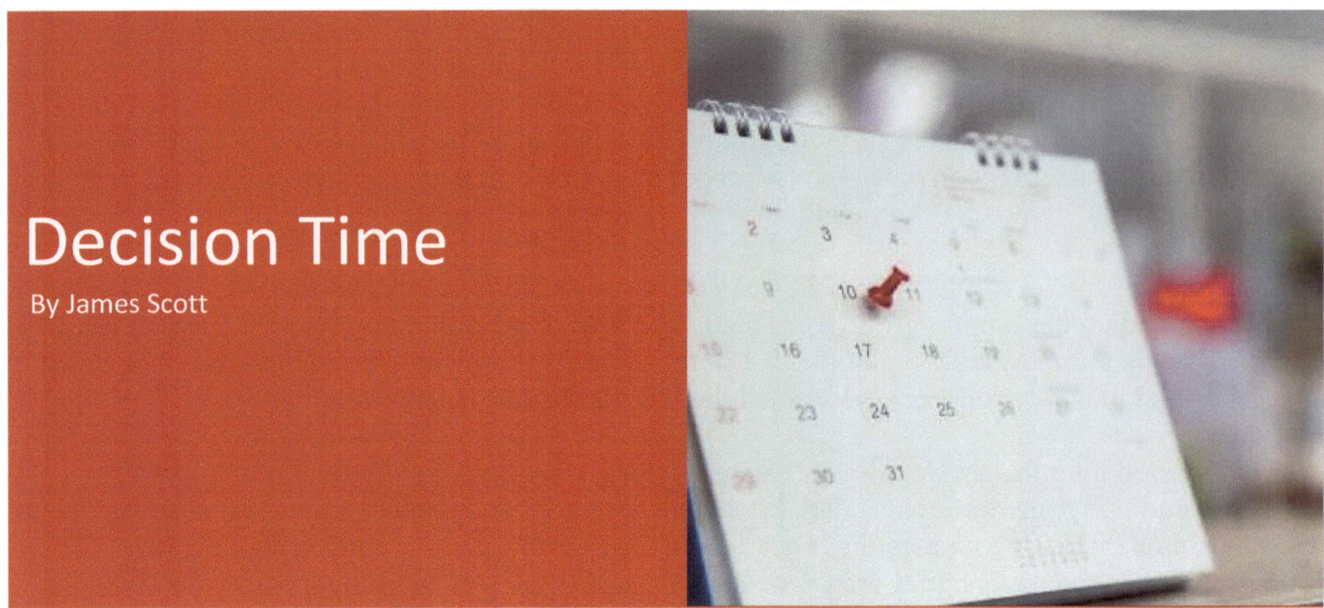

At the risk of sounding dramatic and perhaps taking an overly simplistic view on things in this moment, I believe that brain injured or not, we all must choose between living life on life's terms with, its oftentimes uncomfortable, acceptance, or constant struggle. While the first option with its discomfort, may not seem too appealing, let me assure you the constancy of futile efforts at control of the latter makes intermittent duress seem like a vacation.

As I write these words, the image of my paternal grandfather and namesake playing the violin for me flashes in my minds' eye. Believe me, it is much resistance and attempting to block reality that brings me to this realization. However, as is often the case, after struggling to adjust to the new normal of living in a Covid-19 dominated world combined with the painful experience of having the woman I love decide her life is better without me in it, I'm struggling with acceptance.

> "It's hard to resist judging myself for being immature, or at least developmentally behind my peers for experiencing my first heartbreak at thirty-eight years old."

It's hard to resist judging myself for being immature, or at least developmentally behind my peers for experiencing my first heartbreak at thirty-eight years old. Self-judgement aside, I'm truly devastated. Perhaps, I assumed that past traumas would have conditioned me to better handle this emotional pain, which has proven false. This faulty assumption shouldn't be a surprise to me when I realize that my prior difficulties have always been buffered by alcohol, with my TBI followed by a six week period of minimal consciousness and a lack of understanding of the permanence of my injury. Maybe the individual who stated, "ignorance is bliss", was on to something. But as you hear in the recovery community, "Once you know, you can't not know."

So here I sit, having finished my third hour of Zoom meetings today before noon faced with a choice: Continue to try and mask the pain of seeing the collapse of a relationship I wanted to spend the rest of my life in, or trust that things will be ok. I guess I have to be grateful; grateful for the miracle that I don't want to drink, and for the amazing experience of being a part of an incredible woman and her awesome boy's lives for more than a year. I forget where I heard it, but the saying, "Some days are for chasing our hopes and dreams, and others we just need to put one foot in front of the other", seems pertinent now. I guess for now I'll just focus on moving my feet. A book read by many in the recovering community puts it beautifully: "We were in position where life was becoming impossible, and if we had passed into the region from which there is no return through human aid, we had but two alternatives: One was to go on to the bitter end, blotting out the consciousness of our intolerable situation as best we could; and the other, to accept spiritual help."

> ## "As with most addictions, or almost all unhealthy behaviors for that matter, the problem is generally not the substance or action itself, but rather it represents a presenting symptom of an underlying problem."

As with most addictions, or almost all unhealthy behaviors for that matter, the problem is generally not the substance or action itself, but rather it represents a presenting symptom of an underlying problem. Come to think of it, and I know for myself this to be the case, the underlying "problem" isn't actually the cause of duress. It is a lack of acceptance from which stems all kinds of maladaptive behaviors intended to distract from or mask the friction one feels with reality, or "life on life's terms." So, what exactly is this decision that I just mentioned?

While I really hate to be that guy including so many quotes in his writing as to barely offer any original prose, it is with humility that I recognize nearly any thought I have has been thought before. And what do you know? In this case a quote oft attributed to Buddha concisely describes the choice before me and faced by all of us: "Pain is inevitable, suffering is optional." For it is the attempt to delay, mask, or distract from pain that always leads to suffering. I know that I will be well, that I will heal. I will move forward with that certainly.

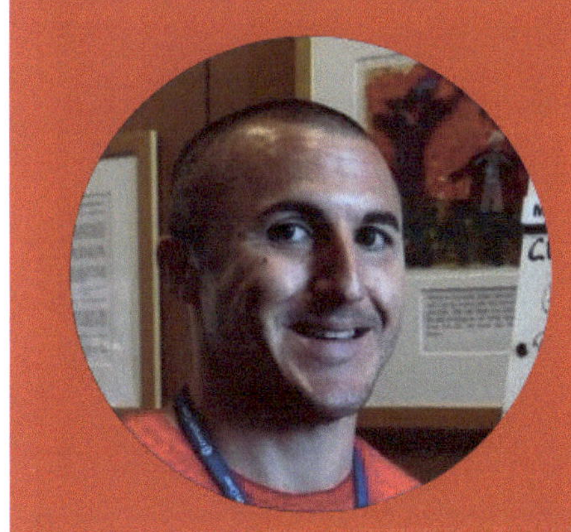

Meet Jim Scott

James sustained a TBI in a motor vehicle crash in July of 2006. Recognizing the cautionary value in his personal story, Jim first began speaking to students with KC's Community Education program. Jim has also worked with Northeast Rehabilitation Hospital's Think First National Injury Prevention Foundation. In 2012, Jim published a memoir titled 'More Than a Speed Bump: Life Before and After Traumatic Brain Injury.'

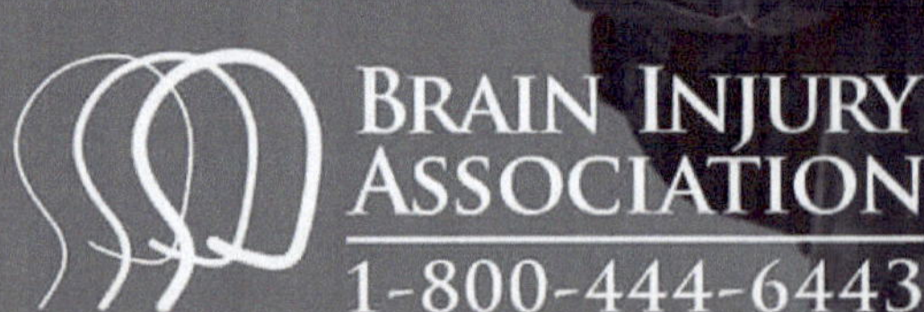
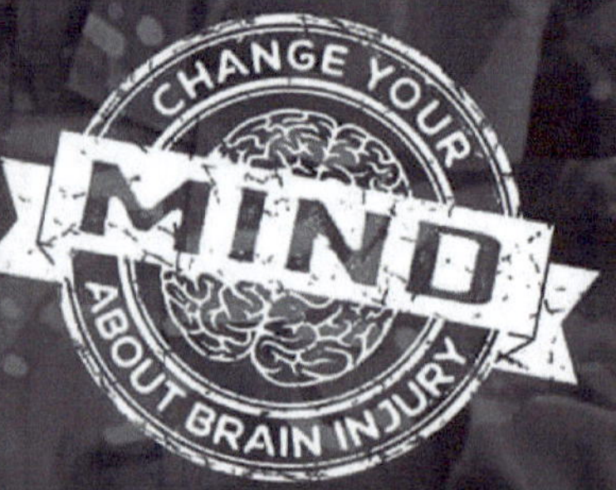

BRAIN INJURY AWARENESS
DID YOU KNOW?
Brain injury changes the way you think, act, move and feel.
#ChangeYourMind
Learn more at www.biausa.org
BRAIN INJURY ASSOCIATION
1-800-444-6443
CHANGE YOUR MIND
ABOUT BRAIN INJURY

Comfortably Numb

By Andrew Davie

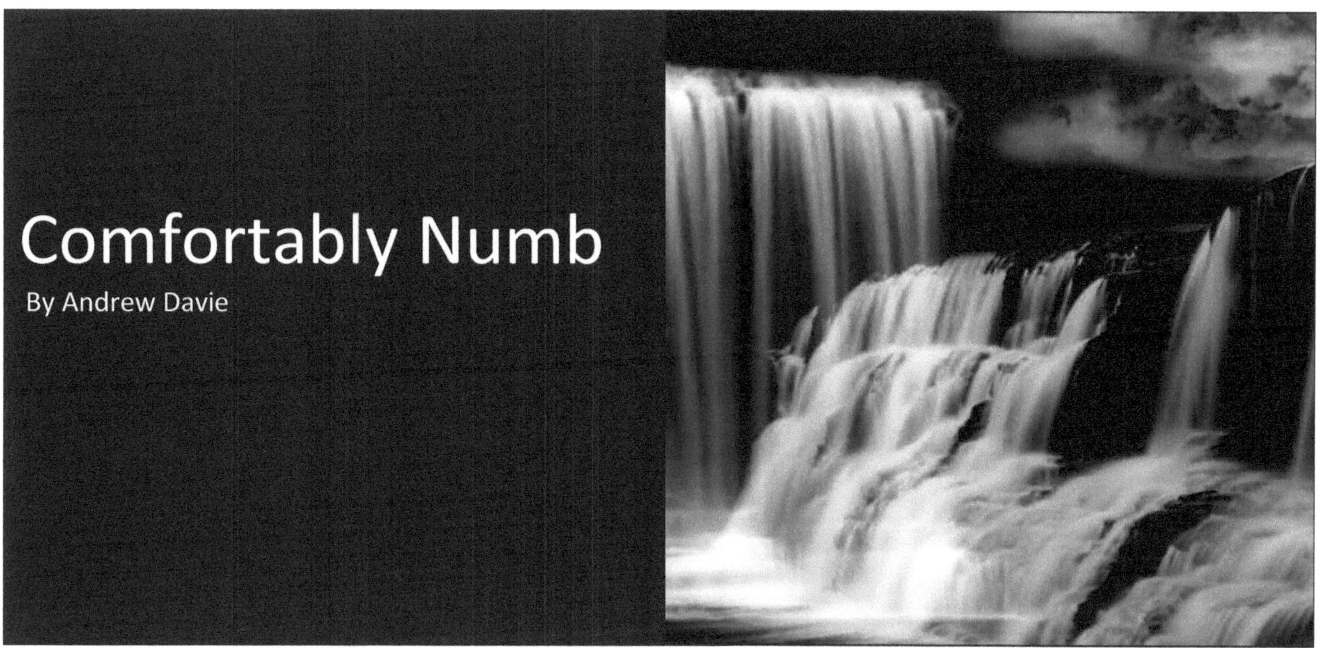

Recovering from a ruptured brain aneurysm hasn't been easy by any stretch, but thankfully most of the physical limitations that still exist are more nuisances than problems. My balance is a little off, and I need to wait for my vision to settle if I move my head. That's about it concerning any lingering physical ailments. However, I have acclimated to these differences and now they are part of my life. The emotional recovery is a little more difficult to adjust to since I have trouble making emotional connections. The euphoria, joy, sadness, etc. I used to feel with experiences aren't there anymore. The uncertainty of whether this will return has been the one obstacle that can be overwhelming.

> "Of course, the pandemic changed the landscape as well. I went from having a difficult unique experience to a difficult universal one."

Of course, the pandemic changed the landscape as well. I went from having a difficult unique experience to a difficult universal one. Most of the progress I had made, and steps I had taken, in terms of going back to work, volunteering, were either canceled entirely or became virtual. Dating, which hadn't been successful, would also be put on hold. The inability to have emotional connections practically made dating moot; although some interesting moments occurred which seemed to be straight from an episode of Curb Your Enthusiasm. For example, do you tell your date you've had a ruptured brain aneurysm? At what point do you bring it up? Does there need to be a segue?

 "Do you want to get an appetizer? By the way…"

Now, along with the continued recovery, due to the pandemic I was faced with spending most of my time alone in my apartment. So, earlier this summer, my mother drove to pick me up and brought me to my parent's house. At least, this way, I was guaranteed human interaction every day. I didn't know how long I would stay with them, but we arrived in mid-June, and I'm still here. I will continue to adjust to everything, though.

During the last two years, there have been many people and organizations who have been helpful both with my recovery and keeping me motivated, such as Brain Injury Services, and I continue to move forward. The recovery process in general reminds me of the chorus from the song "Opposites Attract" by Paula Abdul. "I take two steps forward. I take two steps back. (We come together cause Opposites Attract)." Recovery, as well as many other experiences, tends to move in spirals, and often it seems like you haven't made much progress. One of the helpful mantras which have worked

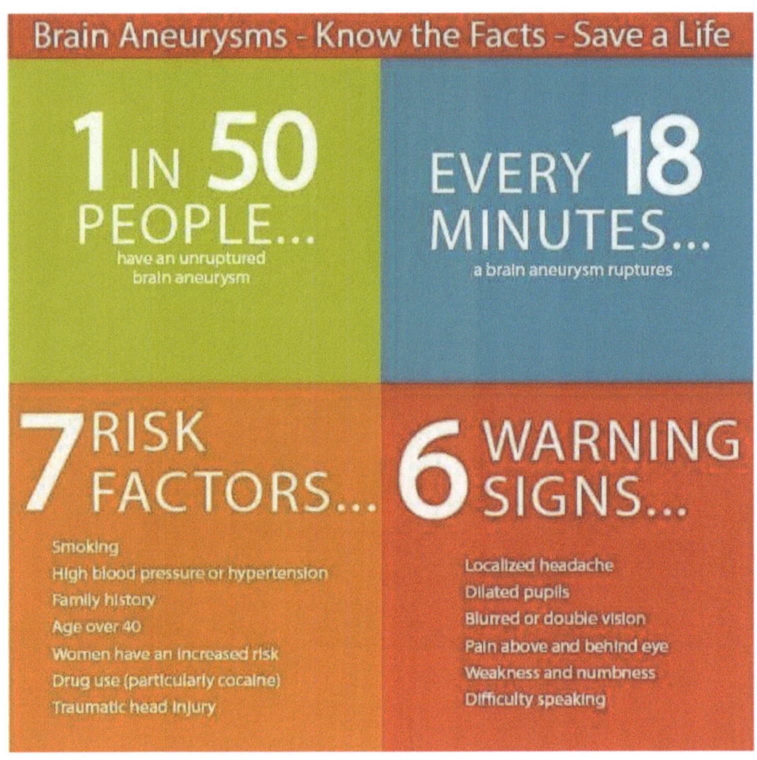

for me to stay level is "Find something purposeful and meaningful to live for each day." If I attempt to consider what the next year, month, or week might look like it can get overwhelming very quickly.

I still sometimes fixate on uncomfortable questions that don't have answers. Will I ever start a family? Is that high on my list of priorities? These questions are all potential pitfalls. Many of them are difficult to contemplate even without a brain injury. Taking it one day at a time, while cliched, has helped tremendously.

My experience with a ruptured brain aneurysm is similar to a passage I read in the book The Tiger, by John Vaillant, about people who've been attacked by tigers and survived. "There are, scattered around the hinterlands of Asia and — increasingly — elsewhere, a small fraternity of people who have been attacked by tigers and lived… very rarely is there anyone in their immediate vicinity who fully appreciates what happened to them out there and, in this way, the lives of tiger attack survivors resemble those of retired astronauts or opera divas: each in their own way has stared alone into the abyss."

Life rarely works out the way we intend. I'm reminded of a quotation from the film Greenberg, in which a disillusioned character is told by a friend something like "You're finally ready to embrace the life you never planned on having." Believe it or not, the film Platoon, about the Vietnam war, has a few quotations that apply to the recovery process; the first "There's the way things ought to be, and there's the way things are." I think about this quotation frequently. The second "All you have to do is make it out of here, and every day the rest of your life is gravy."

However, the most profound quotation which helps me on difficult days was written by Buddhist teacher Prema Chodron, which I'll paraphrase: "Things falling apart is a kind of testing and also a kind of healing. We think that the point is to pass the test or to overcome the problem, but the truth is that things don't really get solved. They come together and they fall apart… the healing comes from letting there be room for all of this to happen: room for grief, relief, misery, and joy."

The Stockdale Paradox, named for Admiral James Stockdale, has also been helpful to keep everything in perspective. He had been a prisoner of war in Vietnam, and what helped him endure and ultimately survive was the following quotation. "You must never confuse faith that you will prevail in the end—which you can never afford to lose —with the discipline to confront the most brutal facts of your current reality, whatever they might be."

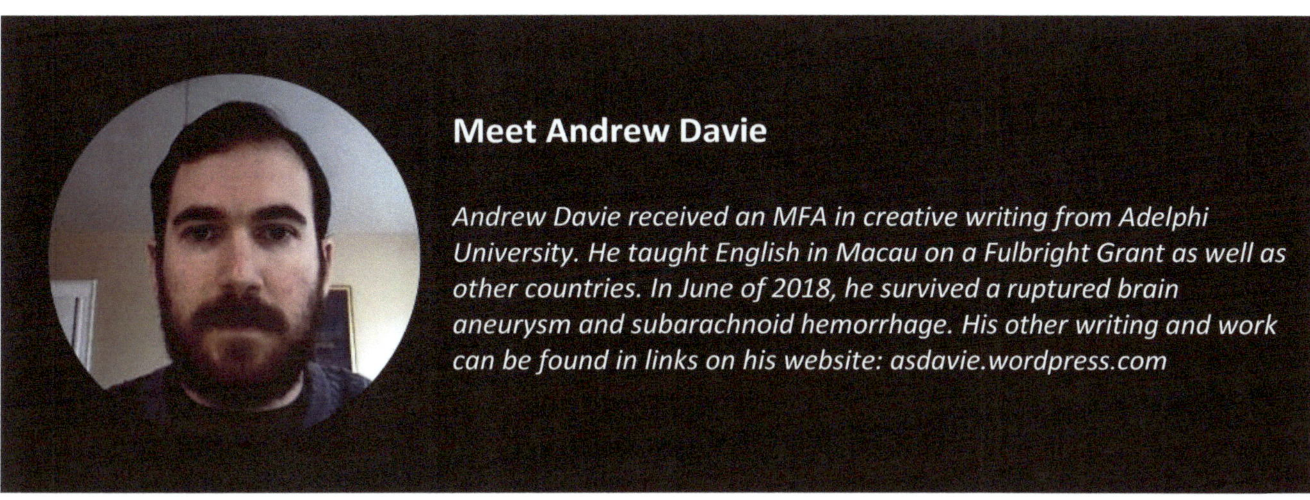

Meet Andrew Davie

Andrew Davie received an MFA in creative writing from Adelphi University. He taught English in Macau on a Fulbright Grant as well as other countries. In June of 2018, he survived a ruptured brain aneurysm and subarachnoid hemorrhage. His other writing and work can be found in links on his website: asdavie.wordpress.com

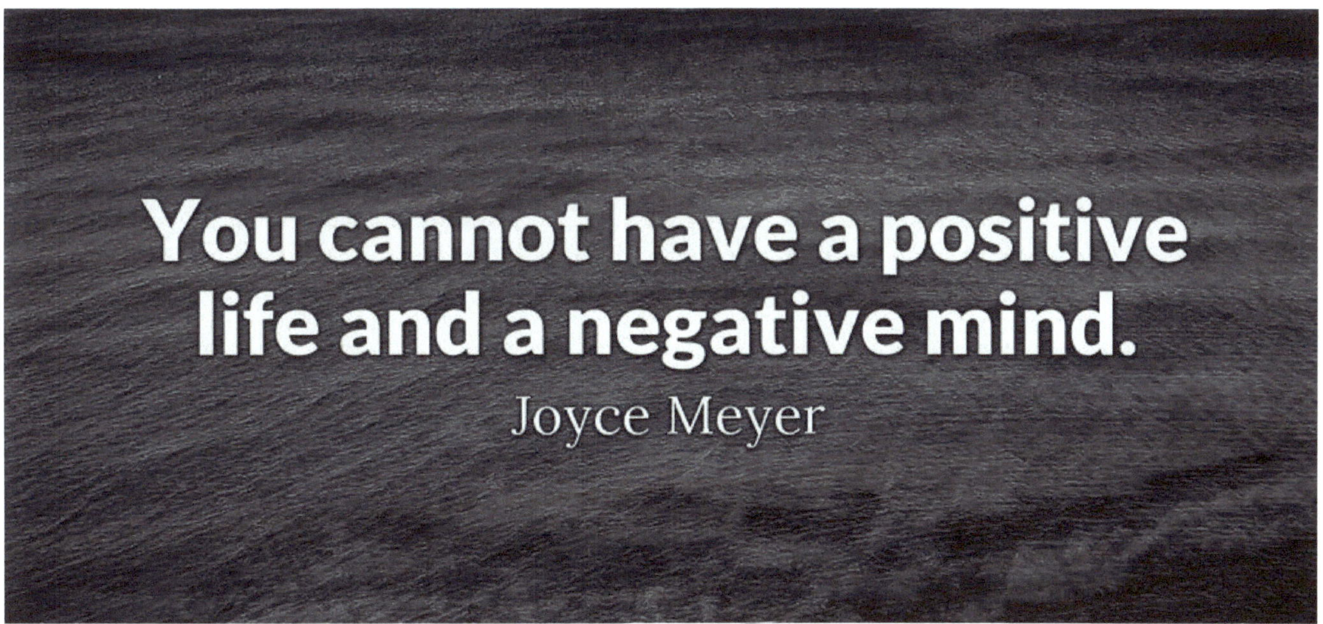

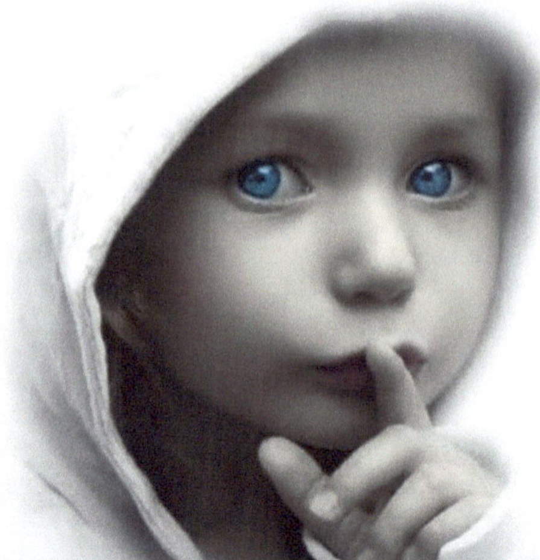

The Paradox of Silence

If I remain silent, my words will not betray me.

If I remain silent, my confusion remains within.

If I remain silent, I won't say something that I regret (again).

If I remain silent, no one can see that I am disabled.

If I remain silent, no one can hear my Soul cry.

If I remain silent, I can walk among the 'uninjured' without drawing attention.

If I remain silent, those who knew me 'before' will see no change.

If I remain silent, I will dwell alone in isolation.

If I remain silent, no one will ever know.

If I remain silent, those who can help me never hear my cries.

If I remain silent, I shut myself off from the love and help of others.

I am destined to never move forward...

If I Remain Silent

Your story has value. Kindly consider submitting your story for publication.

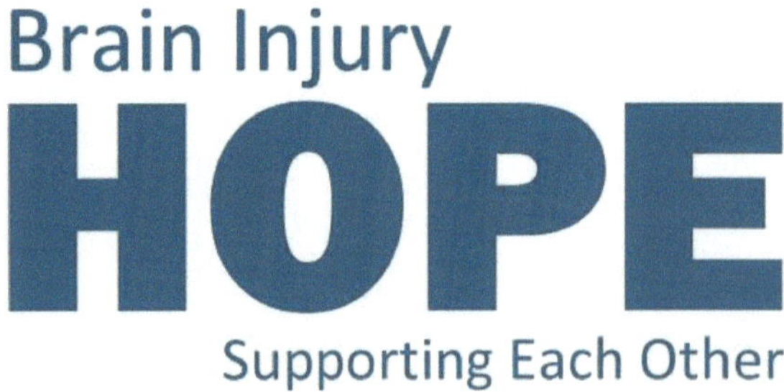

Dear Friend

By Rebecca Veenstra

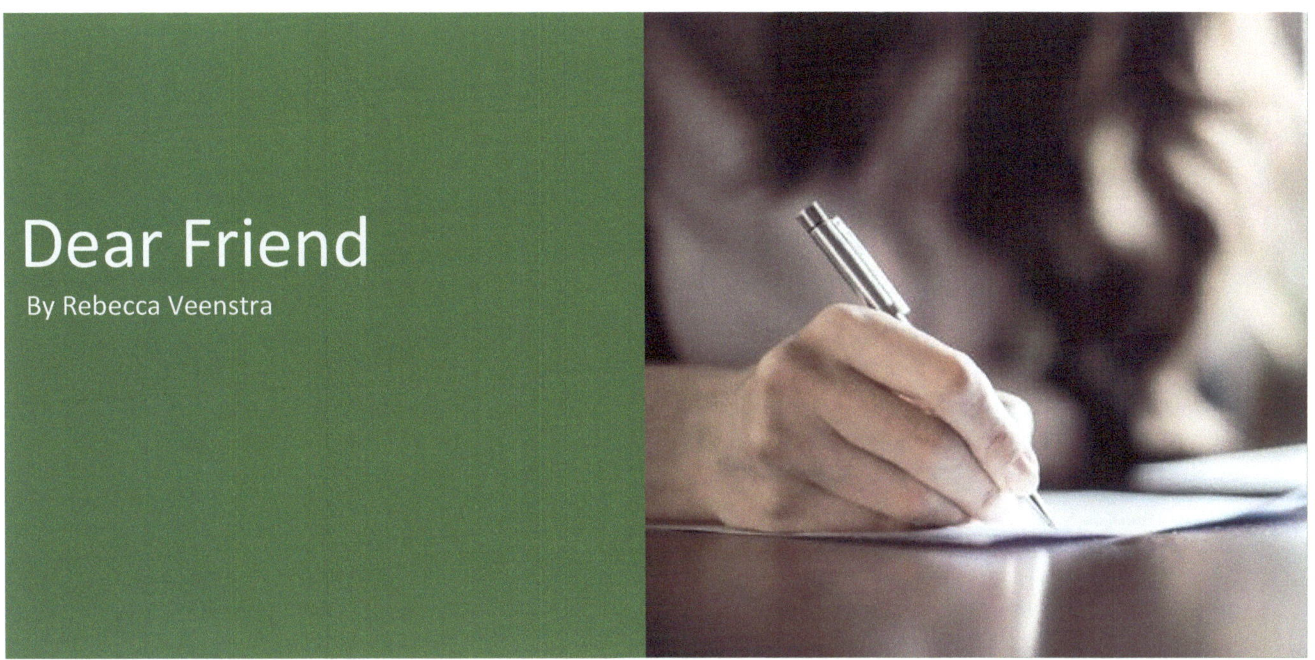

I made a friend who is trying to learn about my TBI. In my attempts to share what it is like to live with an injured brain, I wrote this to my friend…

Dear Friend,

Thank you for reading the webpage I sent you about brain injury. I appreciate that you are trying to understand what I am going through. I am sorry it was confusing yesterday when I asked you not to slam the fridge. I thought the page on hyperarousal on the brain injury website might help to explain.

I now see that there has been a miscommunication. I would like to clear that up if I can, because you seem to think only things that slam are creating the problems in my life. It's not just loud sounds. I mean it is...that's the PTSD. My brain registers a certain frequency of "bang" as danger because the car crash sounded like a bomb going off. Any sound that my brain interprets as similar enough in frequency to the crash sound causes an involuntary muscle movement. That's why things that slam make me jumpy. If I get triggered by bangs repeatedly it "stacks' …adding up. Each involuntary muscle movement is accompanied by a burst of adrenaline. That's what adds up, the adrenaline. So, the jumpiness will be more pronounced over a duration of time until my brain relaxes again. The same adrenal response occurs with sensory overstimulation, which is very different, despite the neurological outcome being similar. The PTSD compounds the overstimulation that results from the TBI damage. They're like Bonnie n Clyde... ganging up on my neurology.

Bright lights, fast movement, music, people talking, any visual or auditory or tactile stimulus, conversation--they can all create a state of neurological hyperarousal. That is experienced as an overload of adrenaline and low cognitive function. Tense, over stimulated neurology and bodily tissues saturated with stimulating hormones. How does neurology relax? I don't know. It takes time.

That's the best I can answer that. I imagine it like a percolation of sorts...the tissues are saturated with adrenaline or the resulting neurotransmitters. The 'duration of time' for this process to conclude is dependent upon how saturated I have become and how long it takes my body to process and move the stimulating chemistry out.

The brain injury website talks about a malfunction of a damaged brain's ability to sort out the stimulus in the environment. The term used is the "brain's filter", which is a perfect description. Think of it like photography. A lens filter takes out the unwanted light information. So, you can view what you want to see. As infants we learn to filter out everything but our mother's face and the sound of her voice. We continue to build our filter throughout our infancy and life. My filter was shattered at 42. My brain was like an infant in its ability to filter six years ago.

Try to perceive your environment next time you are out. I guarantee that if you really sit somewhere for a bit and make yourself separate out all the sights and sounds, you will be astonished at how much you unconsciously disregard every second of the day. A working filter is an amazing thing to behold. I'm amazed at the things people don't notice. I'm actually jealous. Blades of grass in the lawn... really...break it down...it's mind boggling.

Like looking at a bookshelf, you see a shelf of books. My brain wants to know what everything says, the colors of the bindings, the shapes and sizes, the wood of the shelf, the shadows cast. I don't personally have a vested interest in the details.

My brain just can't ignore them. When I was newly injured, I would experience severe nausea from visual and auditory stimulus. My tolerance is greatly improved. Nevertheless, my brain is working double and triple time because the program has glitches to work around. The hardware is damaged. The software has to compensate by working extra hard to get around the damage which translates to extra slow and sensitive. Sensitive in the sense like if you had a computer that was bogged down with too many files it's trying to process simultaneously, and you started trying to upload more files...the more you demand of it the worse the situation gets.

When I say damaged, I mean that my injury is "diffuse." I have what is called shearing. One little area of my brain didn't get hurt. The whole thing did. It's called a coup counter coup injury. Lots of the little fragile neural connections shattered like strands of glass when the truck hit. Then my brain, which is like Jell-O as much as it's like strands of glass, sloshed around in my skull w the impact, shearing off more glass strands from front to back and side to side, with every slosh and bang.

In the first years after I was injured, I could not understand people talking when there was a TV in the background. I could not read words when there was music playing. I would throw up and break into a sweat when therapists put headphones on me w raucous orchestra music playing. Many years later now, I have increased my tolerance a lot. I have come miles and miles.

> **In the first years after I was injured, I could not understand people talking when there was a TV in the background. I could not read words when there was music playing.**

But these past few years since therapy ended have been me learning that it's not over. It's not gone and to hyper stimulate myself, though euphoric initially-- is detrimental to my well-being. Therapy, despite being well intentioned, was a long haul of constant overstimulation between transport, relearning to drive and walk again and the overscheduling. Once it and the accompanying legal battles were over and I had achieved my goals: walking with a cane instead of a walker or sitting in a wheelchair and driving independently with hand controls, I tried to re-enter normal life. I jumped in like I had been away from home for years and wanted to embrace everything that I had been missing at once. I tried to just go along like everything is kosher. I liked the high of loud music, fast driving and being social.

If I just try to power past my struggles, it's like climbing a ladder. With every rung is more distance to fall. The fall is because when the percolation concludes my brain chemistry is off. The high chemicals wear out and I'm left w the brain chemistry of a severely depressed person. After the adrenaline crash/percolation ending, I am low for a few days and then one day I wake up and can say, "I feel a little more human today. I think my bucket might be almost full."

The crashes have come often over the last few years. At first, I would wallow in them as much as I would fight them with noisy songs, pushing myself through them angrily, expecting them to dissipate, to fade away in time. I wanted to exist in the high-functioning period of time when the adrenaline first hits, before it shuts down my cognition and leaves me confused and too hyper to sleep.

I'm now in the process of learning to sort out incoming stimulus by slowly reintroducing activity, music, and people. I have been learning my threshold--the percolation times. Learning is occurring by me being very self-aware and honest with myself. There's nothing I need you or anyone to do or say differently. I don't want to be treated with kid gloves. If I have a need, I will try to communicate it to those around me as best as I can. I can't live with people trying to anticipate and compensate for me. That makes me feel awkward and extremely uncomfortable.

I just want people I love to understand as best as they can what I am up against and to be able to stand by as I muddle thru without taking the reins or trying to navigate for me. I only need you to respect the struggles I have from a place of love and solidarity, not sympathy or pity. I don't want to be coddled. I'm a bad ass and I'll figure out what I can. Probably I'll screw up and fall a lot, but as long as I know I'm loved regardless of how confusing and banged up I might get I'll be ok. It's my journey and I need to learn to teach my loved ones about it.

I hope my commitment to sharing as best as I can, that our friendship will grow from my attempts to be understood by you. I am humbled and grateful for you taking interest and trying to wrap your mind around it all.

I sure do love you tons!

-Rebecca

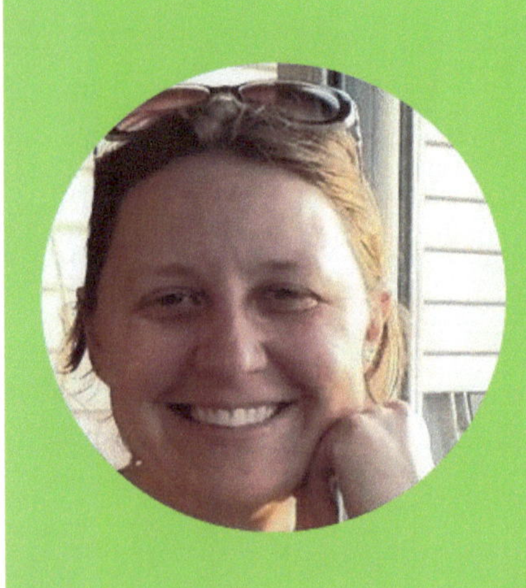

Meet Rebecca Veenstra

"I am 47 years old. I was an herbalist, runner, work out fanatic, health food nut and writer before a run in with a dump truck in 2014 changed my life forever. I live in Northern Michigan with my two Chihuahuas.

I enjoy gardening and photography. This is my first piece of writing since the crash. It feels good to have my words back again. I am beginning to think of ways I can pay back all the kindness and caring I received through my recovery. I hope to someday find a path that gives me the opportunity to advocate for and support others with TBI and PTSD."

The COVID-19 Wildcard

By David A. Grant

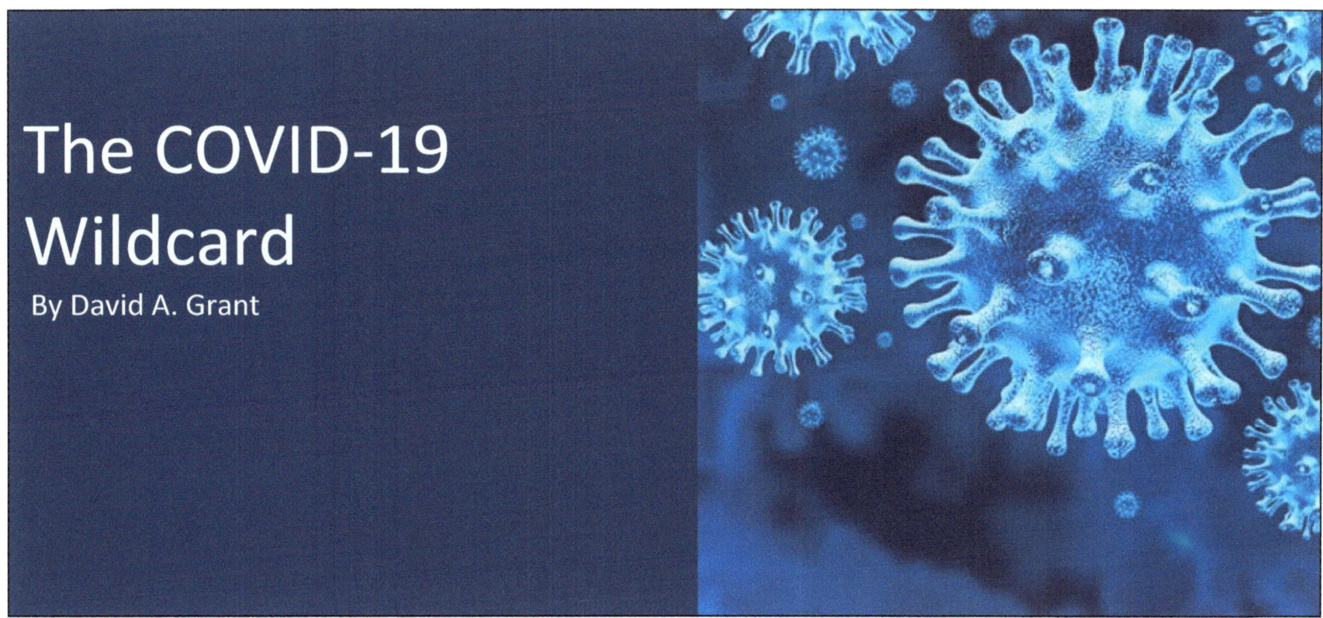

I still find it hard to believe that we have rounded the curve and are now in the second year of a global pandemic. Then again, maybe it's not so hard to believe after all. I'm not the only one who feels like 2020 simply evaporated. Day-by-day, life remained essentially unchanged for Sarah and me. Our weekly grocery delivery was often the only contact we had with the outside world. Being in a high risk category with diabetes, I made the decision very early on not to take any risks.

As 2020 passed, an increasing number of trusted news outlets started to report on the long-term effects of COVID-19. Covid "long-haulers," as they are now called, began to talk about symptoms that sounded all too familiar. I've heard the term "brain fog" more in the last six months than I had in the first decade of my life as a brain injury survivor. Long-haulers spoke of cognitive issues, slower processing times and a level of neuro-exhaustions that defied explanation.

For those of us within the brain injury community, these symptoms are commonplace challenges. But, for the first time, thousands of people, heretofore unfamiliar with brain injury challenges, were living with what sounded like typical symptoms of a brain injury.

In early March, I attended the Congressional Brain Injury Task Force meeting. Thanks to the pandemic, it was a virtual event this year. The topic of this year's meeting was *The Impact of COVID-19 on Persons with Brain Injury.* I attended hoping to learn and to be able to share my new knowledge.

There were a couple of revelations that really came as no surprise. Science has now shown that Coronavirus is a neurotoxin capable of crossing the blood-brain barrier. Simply put, this meant that what has been often called a respiratory illness is now proven to have a neurological component. COVID-19 starves the brain of oxygen. Taking this one logical step further, a brain injury caused by oxygen deprivation is called an anoxic brain injury. Commonly caused by opiate overdoses and drowning, we can now add COVID-19 to the list of brain injury causes.

So what does this mean? Many years ago, when I was a new member of the Brain Injury Association Board of Directors, it was discussed in a meeting that it took the average person five years to reach out to the BIANH for help. Folks tried to go it alone for as long as possible until a desperation point was reached, one where help was needed.

As we move through 2021, and vaccine distribution ramps up, we'll continue to see the rates decline. There has been talk about life looking a little more like it used to as the year progresses, but there is a COVID-19 wildcard that most people haven't given a lot of thought to. As time continues to pass, tens of thousands of people, if not more, will begin to realize that the long-term effects of anoxic brain injury are not simply going to go away.
The big question is this: Are we, as stewards of care, compassion, and concern for those impacted by brain injury, ready for what may be the biggest onslaught of people needing help?

As a society, we will be dealing with the effects of the pandemic for years to come – and for many others, the effects will be lifelong. I just hope we are ready for what's coming.

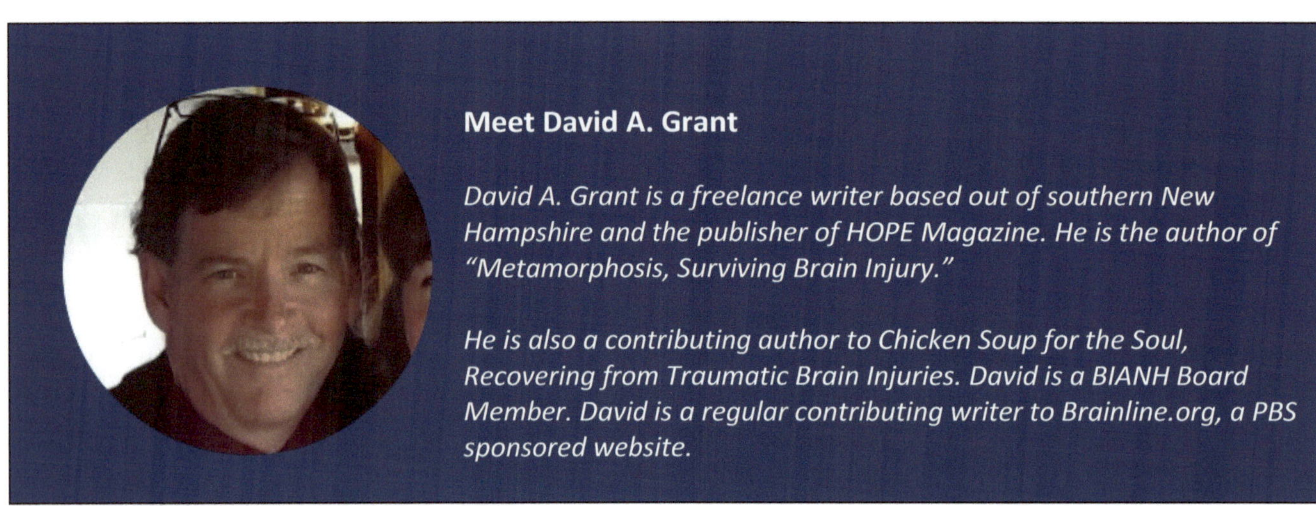

Meet David A. Grant

David A. Grant is a freelance writer based out of southern New Hampshire and the publisher of HOPE Magazine. He is the author of "Metamorphosis, Surviving Brain Injury."

He is also a contributing author to Chicken Soup for the Soul, Recovering from Traumatic Brain Injuries. David is a BIANH Board Member. David is a regular contributing writer to Brainline.org, a PBS sponsored website.

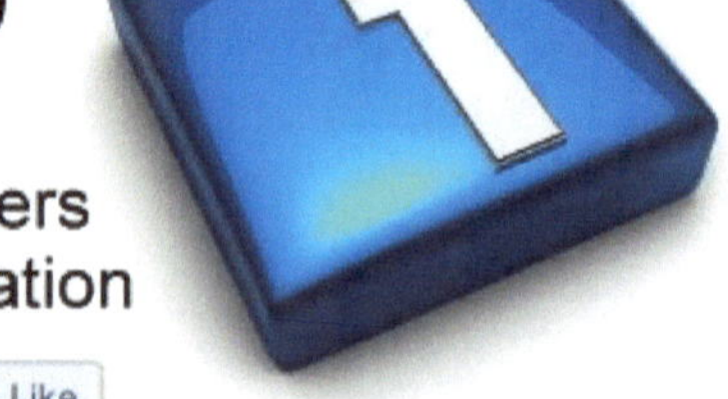

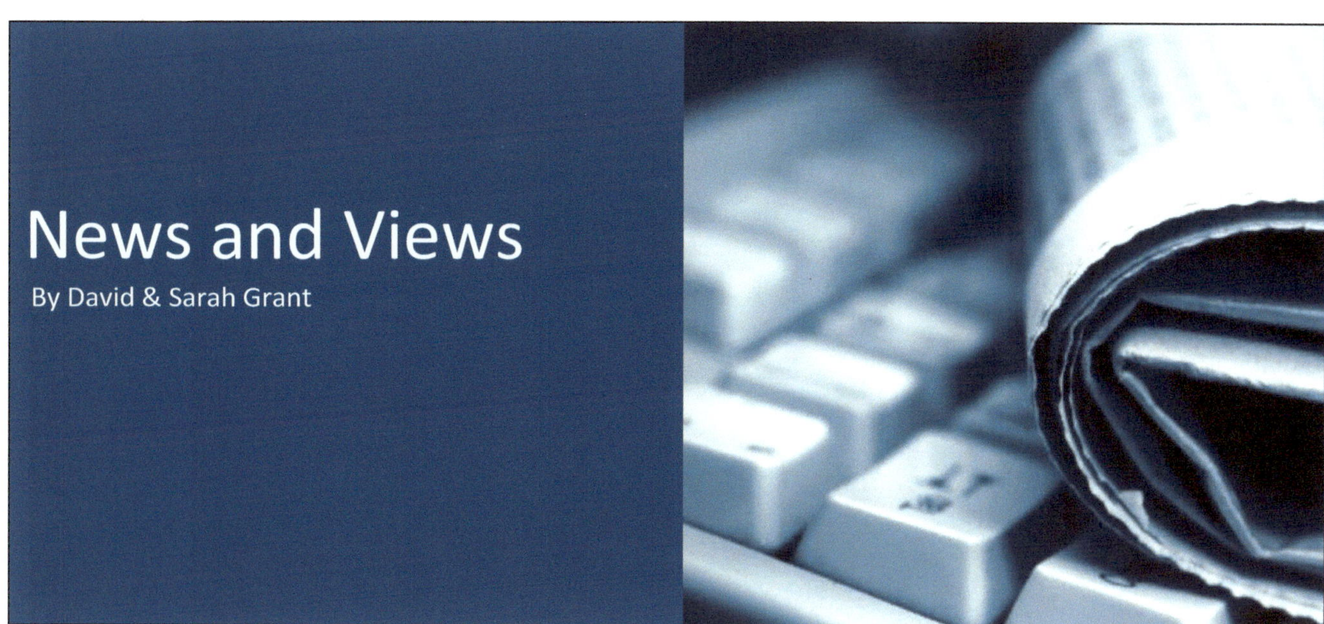

News and Views

By David & Sarah Grant

Brain injury is very much a family affair. A recent question was asked on a brain injury social platform: "What changed after your brain injury?" Comment after comment echoed the same sentiment – everything changed!

For many of us, life is defined as "before and after." Early on after brain injury, it's natural to long for the ease and simplicity of life before everything changed. But brain injury or not, there is no going back. The good news is that there is a way to move forward living with the daily challenges that brain injury brings. Relationships are different, and often stronger. Survivors often develop a level of empathy previously unknown.

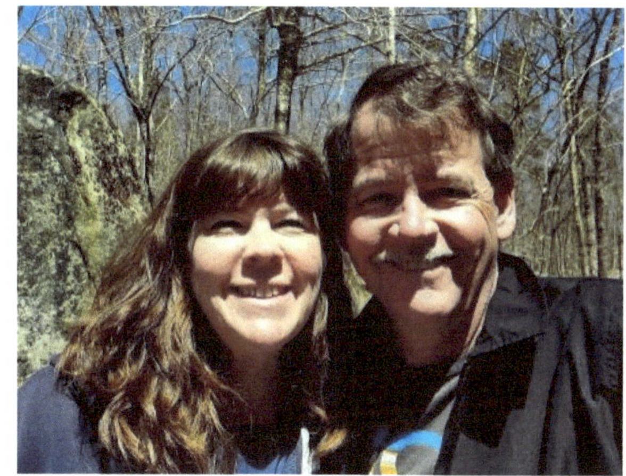

To say that life lately has been a bit stressful would be an understatement of truly epic proportion. The loss of life of the last year has been unfathomable, and with each loss, a family grieves. It's been a heartbreaking journey for so many others.

Our hope for 2021 is that collectively we can take small steps toward healing. If you know of someone who is struggling, use this as a reminder to reach out to them. You might be heling someone more than you ever realize.

~ David & Sarah